The Alkaline Healing Guide: Juices, Herbs, and Natural Cures for Every Ailment

Table of Contents Outline

1. **Introduction: A New Era of Healing**
   - The resurgence of plant-based, natural healing
   - My journey into holistic wellness and the inspiration from Dr. Sebi's research
   - Why juicing and herbs are a powerful combination for disease prevention and healing
2. **Dr. Sebi's Approach to Health and Healing**
   - The alkaline diet: What it is and why it matters
   - Electric foods and their healing properties
   - Detoxification and cellular rejuvenation

- How modern science is catching up with these ancient principles

3. **The Power of Juicing for Health**
   - Why juicing works: Nutrient density and cellular absorption
   - How juicing supports the body's natural detoxification
   - Juicing for energy, skin health, weight loss, and disease prevention
   - Best ingredients for juicing: Alkaline vegetables and fruits
   - Easy juicing recipes for daily vitality

4. **Herbal Healing for Every Ailment**
   - Overview of herbal medicine: Healing with plants from different traditions
   - Top herbs for specific systems in the body (digestive, immune, circulatory, nervous)
   - Herbal remedies for chronic conditions: Diabetes, hypertension, arthritis, and more
   - Herbal teas, tinctures, and tonics: Easy ways to integrate herbs into daily life
   - Dr. Sebi's list of recommended herbs and their benefits
   -

5. **The Science Behind Juicing and Herbal Healing**
   - Phytonutrients and antioxidants: How they combat inflammation and oxidative stress

- Alkalinity and disease: The link between pH balance and health
- Research studies on the healing power of fruits, vegetables, and herbs

6. **Healing with Juices and Herbs: Success Stories**
   - Case studies: How juicing and herbal healing reversed chronic diseases
   - Personal testimonials of transformation
   - Real-world applications of these healing practices

7. **Creating a Daily Healing Routine**
   - How to start juicing and incorporating herbal remedies into your life
   - The best times to juice and take herbs for maximum benefits
   - Creating balance: Juicing, herbs, and a plant-based alkaline diet

8. **Specialized Healing Protocols**
   - Detox protocols: Liver, kidney, and colon cleanses with juices and herbs
   - Anti-inflammatory protocols for autoimmune conditions
   - Juicing and herbs for mental clarity, focus, and emotional balance
   - Hormonal balance: Juices and herbs for women's health

9. **The Future of Natural Healing**
   - How natural healing is becoming more mainstream

- Sustainable healing: Growing your herbs and vegetables
- The role of community and knowledge-sharing in healing journeys

10. **Conclusion: Reclaiming Health Through Nature's Gifts**
    - Empowering yourself with the knowledge of nature's pharmacy
    - Integrating juicing and herbs for long-term health and disease prevention
    - Taking the first steps on your healing journey today

About the Author: JJ Snipes

JJ Snipes passionately advocates holistic health, natural healing, and plant-based nutrition. Drawing inspiration from the groundbreaking work of Dr. Sebi, JJ has dedicated his life to studying the impact of alkaline diets, juicing, and herbal remedies on long-term health and wellness. With a background in wellness coaching and nutritional science, JJ specializes in creating accessible, practical guides that naturally empower readers to reclaim their health.

Known for his compassionate and straightforward approach, JJ believes that true healing is achieved by nourishing the body with natural foods and harnessing the therapeutic power of herbs. Through his best-selling books, workshops, and online platforms, he has helped countless individuals address chronic health issues, boost energy, and embrace an alkaline lifestyle for lifelong vitality.

When he's not writing, JJ experiments with new juice recipes, grows medicinal herbs in his garden, and connects with communities that promote natural wellness. His mission is simple: to educate and inspire others to take control of their health by tapping into nature's healing gifts.

Introduction: A New Era of Healing

Overview: The introduction serves as a primer for readers to understand the shift towards holistic and natural healing practices. Many people return to nature for healing in a world filled with synthetic medicines and processed foods. This chapter establishes the key principles that will guide the reader through the rest of the book: the body's natural ability to heal, the importance of detoxification, and the role of plant-based foods and herbs in promoting health.

Key Sections:

- **The Rise of Natural Healing**: This section delves into the growing movement towards alternative and natural remedies. It introduces the idea that natural healing methods are rooted in ancient practices and are now supported by modern science.
- **Why Juicing and Herbs?** An explanation of why juicing and herbs, when combined, form a powerful duo for healing. Juicing allows for quick nutrient absorption, while herbs provide targeted healing effects.

- **The Body's Ability to Heal Itself**: The body is naturally self-repaired, and given the right tools (proper nutrition, detoxification, rest), it can recover from a wide range of ailments.
- **How to Use This Book**: A brief guide on navigating the chapters and applying what you learn to your healthy journey.

Chapter 1: Dr. Sebi's Approach to Health and Healing

1.1 Who Was Dr. Sebi?

- **Overview**: This section delves into Dr. Sebi's life and philosophy. It outlines how Dr. Sebi's holistic approach—based on alkaline nutrition, plant-based foods, and herbal remedies—challenged conventional medical practices.
    - **Dr. Sebi's Teachings**: Understanding the philosophy behind Dr. Sebi's alkaline diet and how he viewed disease as an imbalance caused by mucus and acidity.
    - **The Legacy of Dr. Sebi**: This book explores how Dr. Sebi's teachings have influenced modern natural healing practices, with testimonials from people whose health has been transformed by following his protocols.

1.2 The Alkaline Diet: A Foundation for Health

- **What Is an Alkaline Diet?** This section explains pH balance and why maintaining an alkaline environment in the body is critical for health. It will highlight how certain foods are acidic while others are alkaline and why eating alkaline foods

helps reduce inflammation and the risk of chronic diseases.
- **Acidic vs. Alkaline Foods**: Detailed lists of acidic foods to avoid (e.g., processed meats, refined sugars, dairy) and alkaline foods to include (e.g., leafy greens, avocados, berries).

1.3 The Importance of Electric Foods

- **Electric Foods Defined**: "Electric foods" refer to natural, unprocessed plant-based foods that provide the body with essential nutrients and minerals. Dr. Sebi emphasized consuming these foods because they are bioavailable and support cellular health.
  - **Top Electric Foods**: A list of the most nutrient-dense, alkalizing foods such as sea moss, nopal cactus, quinoa, watercress, and hemp seeds.
  - **Sea Moss and Its Benefits**: Dr. Sebi recommends sea moss as a key electric food because of its high mineral content and ability to support immune function, thyroid health, and digestion.

1.4 Detoxification and Cellular Regeneration

- **Why Detoxification Matters**: A guide to understanding why the body needs to detoxify and how toxins, heavy metals, and processed foods contribute to disease. This section explains how detoxing aids in reducing inflammation, supporting liver and kidney function, and promoting overall vitality.
    - **Cellular Regeneration**: How alkaline foods and herbs support the body's ability to regenerate damaged cells. The focus is on how detoxification, when paired with proper nutrition, allows the body to repair and rebuild.

Recipes:

- **Alkaline Detox Juice**: A refreshing and detoxifying juice made with cucumber, celery, kale, lemon, and ginger to support the liver and kidneys.
- **Electric Smoothie**: A nutrient-packed smoothie made from mango, sea moss, avocado, and

coconut water to nourish cells and restore energy.

Chapter 2: The Power of Juicing for Health

2.1 Why Juicing is Effective

- **The Benefits of Juicing**: Juicing allows the body to receive a concentrated number of vitamins, minerals, and enzymes without the digestive system breaking down fiber. This quick absorption helps to nourish the body at a cellular level, delivering a high dose of nutrients.
    - **Liquid Nutrition**: Explanation of why liquid nutrition is especially beneficial for those with weakened digestion or those recovering from illness.
    - **Juicing vs. Whole Foods**: A comparison of juicing with eating whole fruits and vegetables, explaining when and why juicing might be more effective.

2.2 The Role of Juicing in Detoxification

- **How Juicing Supports Detoxification**: Juicing enhances the body's natural detoxification processes by providing vital nutrients that support the liver, kidneys, and lymphatic system. Key juice ingredients—beets, parsley, and cilantro—are natural cleansers that help eliminate toxins.
    - **Juicing for Organ Health**: Recipes and advice for juices that target specific

organs, such as liver detox juices with beets and kidney-supporting juices with watermelon and parsley.

2.3 Juicing for Specific Benefits

- **Energy Boosting Juices**: Green juices are packed with chlorophyll, which helps oxygenate the blood and increase energy levels.
    - *Recipe*: **Energy Booster Juice**: Spinach, cucumber, green apple, and lemon.
- **Skin Health**: Juices that provide antioxidants like vitamin C and beta-carotene help detoxify the skin and reduce inflammation, promoting a clearer, more vibrant complexion.
    - *Recipe*: **Skin Glow Juice**: Carrot, apple, ginger, and turmeric.
- **Weight Loss and Digestion**: Juices that support digestion and metabolism are typically low-calorie but high in fiber and water content.
    - *Recipe*: **Metabolism Boost Juice**: Grapefruit, lemon, cucumber, and mint.

2.4 How to Juice for Maximum Results

- **Best Practices for Juicing**: This section will cover the best ways to juice for maximum health benefits, such as juicing in the morning on an empty stomach for better nutrient absorption, using a slow-masticating juicer to preserve enzymes, and consuming juices fresh to retain their nutrients.
    - **Storing Juices**: This section covers how to store juices properly (in airtight containers in the refrigerator) and how to prepare juices in advance without losing their potency.

2.5 Juicing Recipes for Every Need

- **Detox Liver Juice**: Beet, carrot, apple, and lemon to support liver detoxification.
- **Immune-Boosting Juice**: Orange, lemon, ginger, and turmeric to enhance immune function and fight off colds and flu.
- **Anti-Inflammatory Juice**: Pineapple, turmeric, ginger, and black pepper to reduce inflammation and joint pain.

Chapter 3: Herbal Healing for Every Ailment

3.1 The Roots of Herbal Medicine

- **Herbal Healing Traditions**: This section introduces readers to the ancient roots of herbal medicine, focusing on how herbs have been used across cultures to treat common ailments. It discusses the resurgence of herbal healing in modern times as a safe and effective pharmaceutical alternative.
    - **Global Herbal Traditions**: A look at How Traditional Chinese Medicine (TCM), Ayurveda, and Indigenous Herbalism have contributed to our understanding of herbal healing.

3.2 Understanding the Body's Systems

- **Herbs for Specific Body Systems**: This section explains how different herbs support various body systems, from the digestive to the immune system. It explains how herbs can work as tonics (for daily support) or as remedies for specific conditions.

- **Herbs for the Digestive System**: Fennel, peppermint, and ginger are used for digestive support and ease bloating or indigestion.
- **Herbs for Circulatory Health**: Garlic, hawthorn, and cayenne promote heart health and improve circulation.
- **Herbs for Immune System Support**: Echinacea, elderberry, and astragalus boost immunity and prevent illness.
- **Herbs for Nervous System Health**: Ashwagandha, Rhodiola, and chamomile reduce stress and anxiety and support the nervous system.

3.3 Herbal Remedies for Common Ailments

- **Anxiety and Stress Relief**: Herbs like lemon balm, lavender, and chamomile help calm the nervous system and reduce anxiety.
    - *Recipe*: **Calm and Relax Herbal Tea**: Chamomile, lemon balm, and lavender for stress relief.
- **Insomnia and Sleep Disorders**: Valerian root, passionflower, and skullcap are known to promote restful sleep.
    - *Recipe*: **Sleep Aid Tonic**: Valerian root and passionflower tincture to support deep, restful sleep.

- **Hypertension and Cardiovascular Health**: Garlic, hawthorn, and hibiscus are known for their blood pressure-lowering effects.
    - *Recipe*: **Blood Pressure Support Tea**: Hibiscus, garlic, and hawthorn berry tea.
- **Herbs for Inflammation and Pain Relief**: Turmeric, ginger, and Boswellia are powerful anti-inflammatory herbs for treating arthritis and chronic pain.
    - *Recipe*: **Anti-Inflammatory Golden Milk**: Turmeric, ginger, black pepper, and coconut milk.

3.4 Practical Herbal Remedies

- **How to Make Herbal Teas, Tinctures, and Infusions**: This section provides step-by-step instructions on making your own herbal remedies, including how to brew herbal teas, create potent tinctures with alcohol or glycerin, and prepare infusions for stronger effects.

3.5 Dr. Sebi's Favorite Herbs

- **Burdock Root**: Known for detoxifying the blood and treating skin conditions like eczema and acne.
- **Sarsaparilla**: High in iron, used for boosting energy and supporting the blood.

- **Elderberry**: A potent herb for boosting the immune system and preventing colds and flu.

Chapter 4: The Science Behind Juicing and Herbal Healing

4.1 The Power of Phytonutrients

- **What are Phytonutrients:** Explanation of phytonutrients, the natural compounds found in plants that provide health benefits such as reducing inflammation and preventing disease.
    - **Types of Phytonutrients**: Overview of flavonoids, carotenoids, polyphenols, and other phytonutrients, along with their benefits for different ailments.

4.2 Antioxidants and Free Radicals

- **The Role of Antioxidants**: How antioxidants in fruits, vegetables, and herbs help to neutralize free radicals, which cause oxidative stress and lead to chronic disease.
    - **Top Antioxidant Foods and Herbs**: Blueberries, spinach, green tea, and turmeric are foods and herbs high in antioxidants.

4.3 The Role of Alkalinity in Health

- **pH Balance and Disease Prevention**: A deeper dive into how maintaining an alkaline internal

environment helps reduce the risk of chronic diseases like cancer, heart disease, and diabetes. How acidic foods contribute to inflammation and disease progression.
- **Scientific Studies on Alkalinity**: Summaries of scientific research linking an alkaline diet to improved health outcomes, including lower inflammation and reduced risk of chronic illness.

4.4 Scientific Studies Supporting Herbal Healing

- **Adaptogens and Stress**: Research into how adaptogenic herbs like ashwagandha and rhodiola help the body balance cortisol levels and reduce the physical effects of stress.
- **Curcumin and Anti-Inflammatory Effects**: Highlighting studies on curcumin (found in turmeric) and its efficacy in reducing inflammation and pain in conditions like osteoarthritis and rheumatoid arthritis.

Chapter 5: Healing with Juices and Herbs: Success Stories

5.1 Real-Life Transformations

- **Testimonials of Healing**: Real stories of people who have reversed chronic illnesses like diabetes, hypertension, and autoimmune diseases through juicing, herbal protocols, and an alkaline diet.
    - **The Power of Detox**: Stories of individuals who followed detox protocols to clear skin issues, lose weight, or recover from chronic fatigue.

5.2 Overcoming Autoimmune Diseases

- **Case Studies**: Real-world examples of people healing from autoimmune conditions like lupus, multiple sclerosis, and rheumatoid arthritis using herbal and juicing protocols.

5.3 Healing from Diabetes and Hypertension

- **Success Stories**: Detailed stories of how individuals reversed diabetes or normalized blood pressure levels by eliminating acidic foods and incorporating daily juicing and herbal remedies.

5.4 Emotional and Mental Healing

- **Emotional Health**: Stories of people who overcame anxiety, depression, and brain fog by using adaptogenic herbs, mood-boosting juices, and a clean, alkaline diet.

Chapter 6: Creating a Daily Healing Routine

6.1 Designing a Daily Juicing Routine

- **How to Structure Your Day**: This section offers sample daily schedules, including when and what to juice for the best results. It includes morning detox, midday energy boosters, and evening calming juices.

6.2 Incorporating Herbs into Your Daily Life

- **Morning, Afternoon, and Evening Herbal Protocols**: Integrating herbal teas, tinctures, and tonics into your daily routine. Advice on using calming herbs at night, adaptogens during the day, and detoxifying herbs in the morning.

6.3 Combining Juicing, Herbs, and an Alkaline Diet

- **Meal Plan Example**: A sample one-day meal plan that shows how to combine juicing, herbs, and alkaline meals for complete nutrition and healing.
    - *Example*:
        - **Breakfast**: Green juice with sea moss gel and quinoa porridge.

- **Lunch**: Alkaline salad with wild greens, avocado, cucumber, and lemon.
- **Dinner**: Steamed vegetables with quinoa and herbal anti-inflammatory tea.

6.4 Overcoming Common Challenges

- **Staying Consistent**: Advice on how to stick to a juicing and herbal regimen despite a busy lifestyle. Tips for preparing juices and teas ahead of time, setting reminders, and creating a routine that fits your life.
  - **Juicing on a Budget**: How to make juicing and herbal healing affordable by focusing on seasonal produce, growing your herbs, and buying them in bulk.

- Designing **a Daily Routine**

  - **Building a Morning-to-Evening Schedule**: A structured guide for integrating juices and herbs into each part of the day.

- Sample **Schedules for Different Goals**

- **Detox, Energy, and Immune Support Routines**: Sample schedules that address specific health goals.

- Juicing **Schedule**

  - **Best Times for Juices**: Morning detox, midday energy, and evening calming juices explained.

- Incorporating **Herbs into Daily Life**

  - **Daily Teas, Tinctures, and Tonics**: How to add herbal remedies for consistent health support.

- Weekly **Shopping and Meal Prep Guide**

  - **Practical Tips**: Weekly shopping list and preparation tips to simplify the healing journey.

Chapter 7: Specialized Healing Protocols

7.1 Detox Protocols

- **Liver Cleanse Protocol**: Daily beetroot, lemon, and dandelion juice paired with burdock root tea detoxifies the liver and improves digestion.

7.2 Anti-Inflammatory Protocols

- **Arthritis and Chronic Pain Protocol**: Pineapple, turmeric, and ginger juice, along with turmeric and black pepper supplements to reduce joint pain and inflammation.

7.3 Hormonal Balance Protocols

- **Women's Health**: Using Vitex tea, maca root powder, and green juices rich in leafy greens to balance hormones during PMS, menopause, or adrenal fatigue.

7.4 Mental Health and Brain Function Protocols

- **Mental Clarity and Focus**: Beetroot and blueberry juice for brain health combined with Rhodiola and ashwagandha to reduce mental fatigue and support focus.

7.5 Immunity-Boosting Protocols

- **Immune Defense Protocol**: Elderberry syrup, echinacea tea, and immune-boosting juices (orange, lemon, ginger) to strengthen the immune system during flu season.

Chapter 8: The Future of Natural Healing

8.1 The Growing Popularity of Integrative Medicine

- **Integrative Health Trends**: What natural healing methods like herbalism, acupuncture, and nutritional therapy combine with conventional medical treatments in integrative medicine practices.

8.2 Sustainability in Natural Healing

- **Growing Your Herbs and Vegetables**: Tips for creating a Home Garden with medicinal herbs and alkaline vegetables to support a sustainable and self-sufficient lifestyle.

8.3 Community and Knowledge Sharing

- **Healing Communities**: The importance of forming or joining a community of like-minded individuals who share knowledge, recipes, and support on the natural healing journey.

Chapter 9: Conclusion—Reclaiming Health Through Nature's Gifts

9.1 The Journey to Empowerment

- **Taking Control of Your Health**: Empowering readers to take charge of their health journey by embracing natural remedies and simple lifestyle changes.

9.2 Long-Term Health Strategies

- **Maintaining an Alkaline Lifestyle**: Encouragement to continue using juicing, herbs, and an alkaline diet as long-term health strategies rather than quick fixes.

9.3 Taking Action Today

- **Get Started Now**: Simple steps readers can take today to begin their health journey, including shopping lists for basic juices and herbs, a 7-day starter guide, and tips for success.

Appendix A: Dr. Sebi's List of Approved Alkaline Foods

Overview: This appendix includes a detailed list of foods approved by Dr. Sebi that are considered electric, alkaline, and beneficial for health. These foods support detoxification, balance the body's pH, and promote healing at the cellular level. The list is divided into categories, making it easy for readers to plan their meals and incorporate more alkaline foods into their diet.

1. Vegetables

- **Amaranth greens (Callaloo)**: Rich in iron and great for blood health.
- **Bell peppers**: High in vitamin C and antioxidants.
- **Cucumbers**: Hydrating and excellent for detoxification.
- **Dandelion greens**: A natural diuretic, rich in calcium and vitamin K.
- **Kale**: High in chlorophyll, supporting detox and energy.

- **Nopales (Cactus)**: Helps regulate blood sugar and is a rich source of fiber.
- **Okra**: High in folate and fiber, good for digestion.
- **Onions**: Anti-inflammatory and rich in antioxidants.
- **Sea vegetables (Nori, Wakame, Dulse)**: Rich in iodine and minerals that support thyroid function.

2. Fruits

- **Apples**: Packed with fiber and antioxidants, great for digestion.
- **Avocados**: Healthy fats that support cardiovascular health.
- **Bananas (burro only)**: Good source of potassium and resistant starch.
- **Berries (blueberry, raspberry, blackberry)**: High in antioxidants that fight free radicals.
- **Cherries**: Anti-inflammatory, particularly beneficial for joint health.
- **Dates**: Rich in natural sugars, providing quick energy.
- **Figs**: High in fiber, promoting healthy digestion.
- **Mango**: Full of vitamins A and C, supports the immune system.
- **Soursop**: Anti-inflammatory and known for its cancer-fighting properties.

3. Grains

- **Amaranth**: A gluten-free grain high in protein and fiber.
- **Fonio**: A highly nutritious ancient grain with significant protein content.
- **Kamut**: Rich in protein and iron, a good alternative to wheat.
- **Quinoa**: Complete protein, meaning it contains all nine essential amino acids.
- **Teff**: High in iron and calcium, excellent for bone health.

4. Herbs and Spices

- **Basil**: Anti-inflammatory and rich in antioxidants.
- **Burdock Root**: Detoxifies the blood and supports liver function.
- **Dandelion Root**: A powerful detoxifying herb that is excellent for the liver and digestion.
- **Ginger**: Anti-inflammatory, helps with digestion, and reduces nausea.
- **Sarsaparilla**: High in iron, great for detoxification and increasing energy.

- **Thyme**: Antimicrobial, supports respiratory health.

5. Nuts and Seeds

- **Brazil nuts** are high in selenium and essential for thyroid health.
- **Hemp seeds** are complete protein and are rich in omega-3 fatty acids.
- **Sesame seeds**: Rich in calcium and other trace minerals.
- **Walnuts**: High in omega-3 fats, supporting brain and heart health.

6. Oils

- **Coconut oil**: Good source of medium-chain fatty acids (MCFAs), beneficial for brain function.
- **Olive oil (cold-pressed)**: Rich in monounsaturated fats and antioxidants, supporting heart health.
- **Avocado oil**: High in oleic acid, supporting skin health and reducing inflammation.

7. Teas

- **Burdock Root Tea**: Cleanses the blood and promotes liver health.

- **Elderberry Tea**: Supports the immune system and fights off colds and flu.
- **Nettle Tea**: Rich in minerals, great for detoxification, and boosting energy.

Appendix B: Herbal Glossary

Overview: This appendix provides a glossary of common medicinal herbs, explaining their benefits and practical uses. Each herb listed includes key properties, typical applications, and guidance on preparing them for optimal health benefits.

Herbs for Detoxification and Cleansing

1. **Burdock Root**:
    - **Benefits**: Detoxifies the blood, supports liver health, and helps with skin conditions such as acne and eczema.
    - **How to Use**: Burdock root is often used in teas or tinctures. Steep 1 tablespoon of dried burdock root in 1 cup of boiling water for 10-15 minutes.
2. **Dandelion Root**:
    - **Benefits**: A natural diuretic that helps cleanse the liver and promote healthy digestion.

- **How to Use**: It can be brewed as tea or added to salads. Add 1 teaspoon of dried dandelion root to hot water and steep for 10 minutes.
3. **Milk Thistle**:
    - **Benefits**: Protects the liver and helps regenerate liver cells.
    - **How to Use**: Milk thistle is often taken as a supplement or tincture. You can also brew the seeds into a tea by crushing them and steeping them in hot water.

Herbs for Immune Support

1. **Elderberry**:
    - **Benefits**: Known for its antiviral properties, elderberry is particularly useful for colds and flu.
    - **How to Use**: Elderberries are often used as syrup, but they can also be brewed into tea by steeping 1 tablespoon of dried elderberries in boiling water for 15 minutes.
2. **Echinacea**:
    - **Benefits**: Boosts the immune system and helps shorten the duration of colds.
    - **How to Use**: Echinacea is often made into tinctures or teas. To use it, boil 1 tablespoon of dried echinacea in water for 10 minutes.

3. **Astragalus**:
    - **Benefits**: Strengthens the immune system and improves overall vitality.
    - **How to Use**: Dried astragalus is commonly used in soups, teas, and tinctures. Add it to soups or make tea by steeping 2 tablespoons in hot water for 15 minutes.

Herbs for Inflammation and Pain Relief

1. **Turmeric**:
    - **Benefits**: Anti-inflammatory and antioxidant, turmeric is effective for arthritis and joint pain.
    - **How to Use**: It is best absorbed when combined with black pepper. Use it in teas and tinctures, or add it to soups and smoothies.
2. **Ginger**:
    - **Benefits**: Anti-inflammatory, helps with digestion, and reduces nausea.
    - **How to Use**: Ginger tea can be made by slicing fresh ginger and simmering it in water for 10-15 minutes.
3. **Boswellia**:

- **Benefits**: Known for its ability to reduce inflammation and alleviate arthritis pain.
- **How to Use**: Often taken as a supplement or tincture.

Herbs for Mental Clarity and Stress Relief

1. **Ashwagandha**:
   - **Benefits**: An adaptogen that helps reduce stress and improve focus.
   - **How to Use**: Ashwagandha is often taken in powdered form, as a tincture, or in capsules. Add 1 teaspoon of ashwagandha powder to smoothies or tea.
2. **Rhodiola**:
   - **Benefits**: Enhances mental clarity, reduces fatigue, and improves stress response.
   - **How to Use**: It is typically taken as a tincture or supplement. For an energy boost, add it to morning tea.
3. **Chamomile**:
   - **Benefits**: Promotes relaxation, improves sleep, and reduces anxiety.
   - **How to Use**: Brew dried chamomile flowers in hot water for 5-10 minutes for a calming tea.

Appendix C: Additional Resources

Overview: This appendix includes a curated list of books, documentaries, websites, and other resources on juicing, herbal medicine, and holistic health for readers looking to explore natural healing in more depth.

Books

1. *Healing with Whole Foods* by Paul Pitchford: A comprehensive guide on the healing power of plant-based foods and herbs.
2. *The Detox Miracle Sourcebook* by Dr. Robert Morse: An in-depth look at the body's detoxification systems and how to use foods and herbs to heal.
3. *The Encyclopedia of Herbal Medicine* by Andrew Chevallier: A detailed reference on medicinal plants and herbs for healing various ailments.

Documentaries

1. *Forks Over Knives*: This documentary explores the health benefits of a plant-based diet and the link between diet and disease.
2. *Fat, Sick & Nearly Dead*: A documentary about one man's journey to regain his health through

juicing, inspiring many to start juicing for their health transformation.
3. *The Magic Pill*: Focuses on the power of real, unprocessed foods to prevent and reverse chronic diseases.

Appendix D: Frequently Asked Questions

Overview: This appendix answers common questions about juicing, herbal healing, and following an alkaline diet. It offers practical tips and clarifications to ensure readers have all the information they need to succeed on their health journey.

Juicing Questions

1. **How often should I juice?**
    - It depends on your goals. You may want to juice daily for detoxification, but 3-4 times a week is effective for general health.

2. **Can I store my juice, or should I drink it immediately?**
    - Fresh juice is best consumed immediately to preserve nutrients, but it can be stored in an airtight container in the refrigerator for up to 24 hours.
3. **What type of juicer should I use?**
    - A slow-masticating juicer is ideal because it preserves more enzymes and nutrients than centrifugal juicers.

Herbal Healing Questions

1. **How long should I take an herbal remedy before seeing results?**
    - It depends on the herb and the condition. Some herbs may offer immediate relief (such as ginger for nausea), while others, like adaptogens, may take several weeks to show full effects.
2. **Can I take multiple herbs at once?**
    - Yes, many herbs work synergistically. However, consult with an herbalist or healthcare professional to avoid interactions, especially if you're on medication.
3. **Are herbs safe for children or pregnant women?**
    - Some herbs are safe, but others may not be suitable. Always consult with a

healthcare provider before giving herbs to children or using them during
- pregnancy.

Alkaline Diet Questions

1. **Can I eat cooked foods on an alkaline diet?**
    - Yes, but the focus should be on whole, unprocessed, plant-based foods. Raw foods are highly recommended, but some steamed or lightly cooked vegetables are also acceptable.
2. **Is it okay to have cheat meals occasionally?**
    - For optimal results, stick to an alkaline diet, but having occasional non-alkaline foods is a personal choice. Balance is key to long-term success.
3. **How do I transition to an alkaline diet?**
    - Start by gradually replacing acidic foods (like dairy and processed grains) with more alkaline foods (like leafy greens and fruits). Make one or two changes at a time to ease the transition

Epilogue: A Personal Journey of Healing Through Juicing

As I close this book, I want to share something deeply personal: how juicing has transformed my life and my mother's health. Like many of you, I initially turned to juicing out of curiosity. But over time, it became clear that this practice was more than a health trend—it was a path to genuine healing.

My mother and I both faced our own health struggles. She had been dealing with high blood pressure and joint pain for years while I battled with low energy and digestive issues that seemed impossible to resolve. Watching her face these challenges with limited relief was difficult, and I felt a profound need to find something that could help us both.

Juicing entered our lives almost by chance, but it quickly became a cornerstone of our daily routines. Starting each morning with a green juice or a detoxifying blend did more than provide nutrients—it gave us energy, clarity, and a renewed sense of vitality. Slowly, my mother's blood pressure stabilized, her joint pain lessened, and she found herself moving with more ease and comfort. Meanwhile, I experienced greater mental clarity, a calmer digestive system, and a sense of wellness I had never known.

This journey has been one of discovery, patience, and genuine connection. Juicing has helped us overcome physical challenges and deepened our bond as we explored recipes, shared new favorites, and celebrated each other's health wins along the way. It's been a transformative experience, reminding me daily of the body's ability to heal when given the right support.

This book inspires you to discover your path to healing. May you find the same peace, energy, and health that juicing has brought to my mother and me. Remember, the journey is unique to each of us, but with nature's gifts on your side, every step is toward a healthier, more vibrant life.

Made in the USA
Coppell, TX
06 July 2025